MW01230792

HEALTHY, QUICK & EASY SMOOTHIES

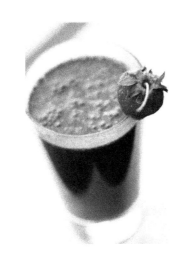

+100 NO-FUSS SMOOTHIES IDEAS YOU CAN MAKE WITH LESS THAN 5-INGREDIENTS FOR WEIGHT LOSS & YOUR WELL-BEING

CHLOE' PITT

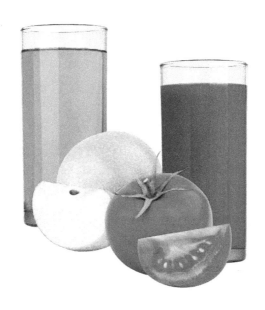

TABLE OF CONTENTS

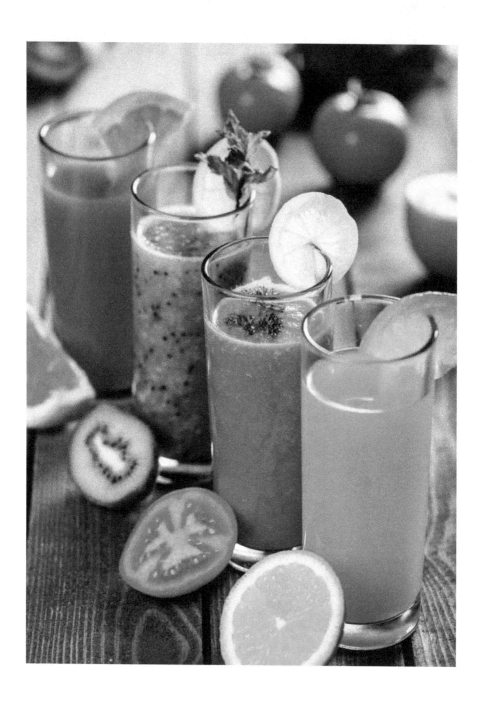

Smoothies are thick and creamy drinks usually mixed with fruits, vegetables, juices, yogurt, nuts, seeds, and/or dairy or non-dairy milk. Drinking a smoothie as the first meal in the morning is a great way to give energy to the body. It also allows you to feel regenerated and purified especially if you want to burn high-calorie foods and foods with refined sugars consumed in the previous

days.The simplest smoothie starts with two essential ingredients: a base and a liquid. From there, you can combine the ingredients to your liking.Many smoothies include frozen produce or ice cubes to give the final product the cool, icy texture of a smoothie. However, their flavor profiles vary greatly depending on the ingredients.Many people consume smoothies as a morning meal or afternoon snack. They can be a great way to incorporate more healthy foods into your diet.Can help increase your intake of fruits and vegetables Smoothies made primarily from fresh or frozen produce can increase your consumption of fruits and vegetables, which provide a diverse range of essential vitamins, minerals, fiber and antioxidants.Together, these nutrients can reduce inflammation, improve digestion and lower the risk of chronic conditions such as heart disease, osteoporosis, obesity and age-related mental decline .

A breakfast staple for many, smoothies can fit into your **meal plan** as a snack, dessert, or an entire meal depending on what you add. A simple **smoothie recipe** is one of the easiest, quickest, and most picky-eater-pleasing way to add a serving (or several) of produce to your diet. Plus, we're learning more about **anti-inflammatory smoothie ingredients** that mean smoothies at home can be an even bigger boost to your overall health. If you're one who doesn't like to drink your food, get your spoon ready and try making a smoothie bowl for a longer-lasting eating experience. Whichever route you prefer, break out your blender and prepare to design your perfect recipe.

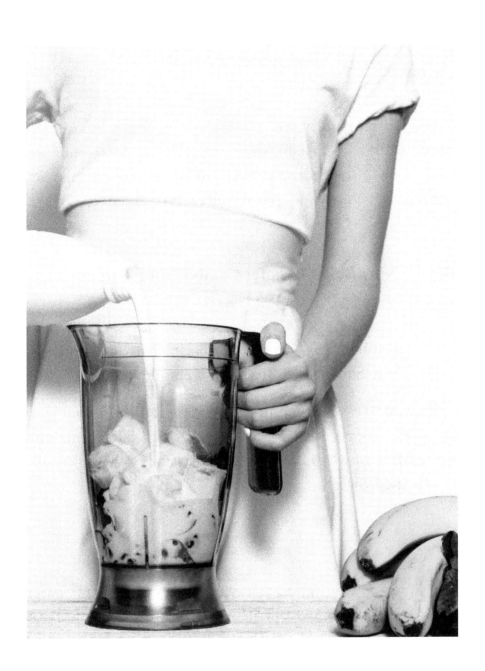

How to Make a Smoothie Step-by-Step

Calling all creative types! There are very few rules when it comes to how to make a smoothie at home. Just about any fruit works, so choose based on your favorite flavors, seasonality, and any food intolerances or preferences.

Buy It: NutriBullet Blender Combo ($140, **Target**)

Just remember this simple formula: Fruit + Juice + Dairy/Dairy Substitute + Ice = Easy Smoothie Recipe Win.

Follow our Test Kitchen pro tips below to design your own smoothie recipe, then learn how to transform it into a **smoothie bowl** and how to give it an über-rich and creamy consistency. Sweet!

Step One: Choose the Fruit

OBVIOUSLY, PICKING THE FRUIT IS AN ESSENTIAL PART OF HOW TO MAKE A FRUIT SMOOTHIE. FOR TWO SERVINGS OF YOUR CUSTOM SMOOTHIE RECIPE, MEASURE 2 CUPS PEELED AND SLICED FRUIT INTO YOUR BLENDER. FEEL FREE TO MIX FRUIT FLAVORS OR STICK TO JUST ONE FAVORITE. (BY THE WAY, LEARN WHICH FRUITS TO STORE IN THE FRIDGE AND WHICH TO LEAVE ON THE COUNTER

How to Make a Smoothie with Frozen Fruit: When fruits are ripe, ready, and in season, **freeze them** (unwashed, sliced, and pitted if necessary) in 2-cup portions in freezer bags to use when they are not so plentiful. Fruit can be frozen up to 9 months. Alternatively, you can purchase frozen fruit at the supermarket to use in your smoothies at home. Replace fresh fruit with frozen in equal quantities.

Step Two: Add the Liquid and Dairy

For the liquid in your smoothie recipe, use 1 cup of:

- Fruit juice

- Juice blend

- Coconut water

- Water

Then add 1 cup of:

- Milk or **dairy-free milk** substitute (plain or flavored)

- Yogurt (plain or flavored)

- **Kefir**

- Buttermilk

How to Make a Smoothie Without Yogurt or Dairy: Omit the dairy element and increase the fruit and juice by ½ cup each.

Step Three: Optional Add-Ins to Make a Smoothie Thicker

Just like at the smoothie shops, you can add bonus bulk-ups to make the consistency of your smoothie more luxurious and offer additional satisfying protein and fiber. Try these:

- ¼ cup protein powder or another powdered supplement

- 1 to 2 teaspoons wheat germ or flaxseed

- ¼ cup silken tofu

- ¼ cup cooked white beans or chickpeas

- 2 tablespoons nut butter (check out this **Protein-Packed Smoothie recipe** for inspiration)

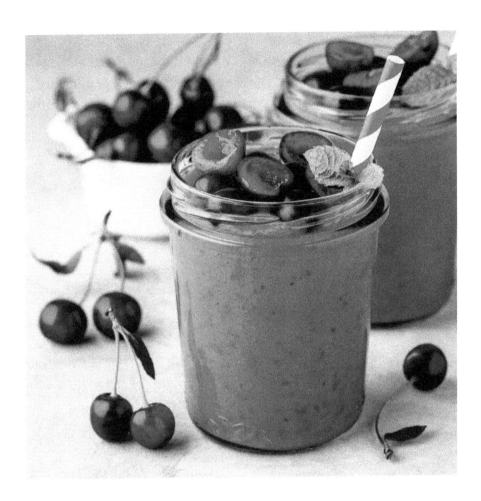

The amount of ice you use depends on how thick you want your smoothie recipe to be. Start with about 1 cup crushed ice for a fairly thick smoothie that is still drinkable with a straw. Omit the ice if using frozen fruit or if you want the smoothie to be thinner and less cold. Cover and blend until nearly smooth. (Then use these tricks to clean a blender in a flash.) Pour into a cup or thermal to-go drink container and slurp up every last drop.

1.Helps You Lose Weight

Smoothies can help you lose excess body weight without skipping any meals. The fruits and berries that are used to prepare these drinks serve as excellent companions for keeping you healthy and feeling cooler on a hot summer morning. The enzymes present in several fruits help dissolve body fat and clear up your circulatory system.

2.Prevents Dehydration

Water is the most abundant thing both on earth and in your body. About 70 percent of your body is water. Having smoothies along with breakfast is a great way to replenish the loss of water in your body during the summer.

3.Makes You Feel Full

People trying to lose weight often skip the morning meal and end up snacking on food in larger amounts between meals. To avoid this, experts advise having smoothies made of excellent fruits and flavors so that you stay full for a long time.

4.Controls Cravings

Smoothies are full of nutrients and flavor. They are an essential part of the best breakfast, as they provide a power-packed start for the day. A lot of protein along with many nutrients subdue food cravings and keep you away from eating junk food.

5.Aid In Digestion

Green smoothies that contain a lot of green leafy vegetables add essential vitamins and minerals to breakfast and aid in digestion. The fiber supplied by these drinks multiplies the benefits of having a delicious breakfast, especially during the summer.

6.Source of Antioxidants

Green tea is a famous source of antioxidants. You can add matcha green tea powder to make your smoothies rich in antioxidants, and these will help prevent a lot of diseases. Grapes, berries and sweet potatoes are natural sources of antioxidants.

7.Enhances Immunity

Immunity refers to the ability of your body to fight against pathogens and diseases. This natural potential becomes degenerated due to several reasons. Interestingly, having smoothies made of ingredients that include nutrients like beta-carotene helps boost your immune system.

8.Curbs Sleep Disorders

People belonging to different age groups around the world often face issues related to lack of sleep and restlessness. A healthy breakfast accompanied by a smoothie made of bananas, kiwi and oats provides calcium and magnesium in good amounts. This induces sleep and helps maintain healthy sleeping patterns.

9.Improves Skin

As you may know, food containing carotenoids, like mango and pumpkin, are highly beneficial for skin and complexion. Therefore, smoothies that contain these ingredients help you keep glowing in the summer.

10. Provides Liquid Food Benefits

Health and nutrition experts worldwide suggest consuming liquid food for better digestion. Smoothies contain blended fruits and vegetables in liquid form that make it easier for the body to break them down.

11. Detoxifies the Body

Foods like garlic, papaya and beets help cleanse your blood and get rid of several toxins accumulated in your body tissues. Thus to have a great breakfast you should include smoothies as reliable detoxifying drinks every day.

12. Boosts Brain Power

It is quite evident that that certain fruits and vegetables increase brain power and boost memory. Mental alertness and concentration is greatly enhanced by ingredients like coconut that are rich in omega-3 fatty acids. Smoothies with these ingredients help the brain work faster.

13. Controls Mood Swings

Organic fruits and vegetables serve as excellent stress busters. Smoothies made of fresh ingredients relieve stress and help you stay happier and healthier.

14. Fights Depression

Fresh vegetables and fruits that are rich in folic acid, like broccoli, spinach and bananas, help keep depression at bay. Patients suffering from depression are advised to eat healthy breakfasts, and smoothies can be very helpful for them.

15.Supplies Calcium

A regular intake of calcium in the right amount is essential for bone and tooth health. Moreover, it can affect hair growth and heart functioning too. Smoothies prepared with dairy or fortified dairy alternatives serve as great sources of calcium for the body.

16.Checks the Growth of Carcinogens

The growth of cancer-causing factors, or carcinogens, can be checked by controlling the growth of free radicals in the body. Fruits like strawberries, blueberries and grapes are rich in antioxidants that inhibit the growth of cancer-causing free radicals.

17.Provides a Good Amount of Fiber

The most common problem people suffer from today is related to upset bowels. A good amount of fibrous food is essential for regulating the excretory system so that you can enjoy summer without worrying about your health. Smoothies with a lot of fruits and vegetables help keep your bowels functioning smoothly.

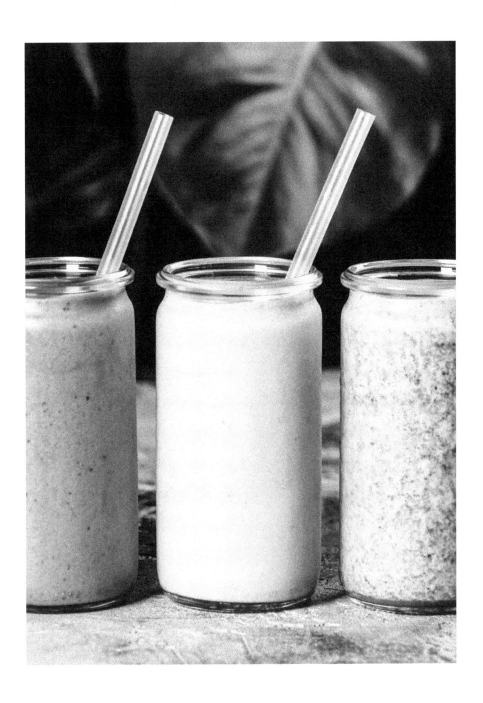

Smoothie recipes

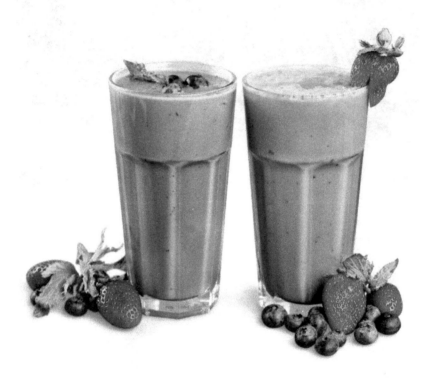

GLEAMING GREEN SPINACH AND LETTUCE SMOOTHIE

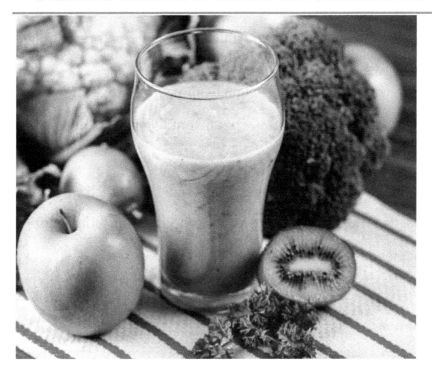

INGREDIENTS

- 3 cups chopped romaine lettuce (or about 1 head)

- 2 cups chopped spinach leaves (about half of a large bunch) ½ cup sliced celery

- ½ cup diced apples (about ½ medium sized whole)

- ¼ cup diced pear (about 1 medium sized wholes)

- ½ cup sliced banana

- ½ tablespoon fresh lemon juice 1 cup water

DIRECTIONS

1. Wash all vegetables and fruits thoroughly before handling them.

2. Put romaine lettuce, spinach and water together in a blender. Process at low speed until mixture becomes smooth.

3. Add celery, apple and pear. Blend mixture at high speed.

4. Lastly, add the banana and lemon juice and puree until well blended. 5. Pour into glasses and serve fresh.

Variation:

ADD ½ CUP EACH OF PARSLEY AND CILANTRO FOR AN EVEN GREENER SMOOTHIE. USING STEMS ARE OKAY, BUT CHOP THEM SO THEY DO NOT RUIN YOUR BLENDER OR SMOOTHIE MAKER.

BOOSTER SPINACH GREENS SMOOTHIE

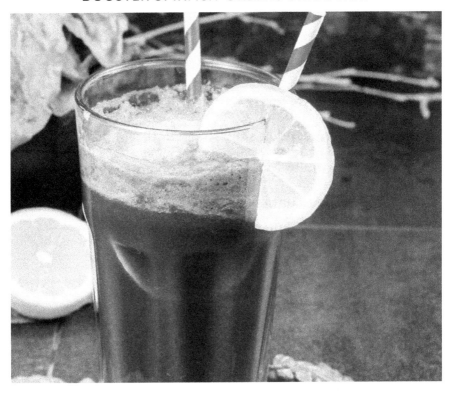

INGREDIENTS

- 1 cup fresh spinach

- 1 cup fresh collard greens

- 4 whole medium sized oranges 3 cups pineapple chunks

DIRECTIONS

1. Squeeze out the juice from the oranges. Use this fresh juice as liquid base for blending the spinach and collard greens together. Blend at slow speed until smooth.

2. Add the pineapples to the orange and greens mixture and blend at high speed until well mixed.

3. Pour and serve immediately.

MINTY PAPAYA GREEN SMOOTHIE

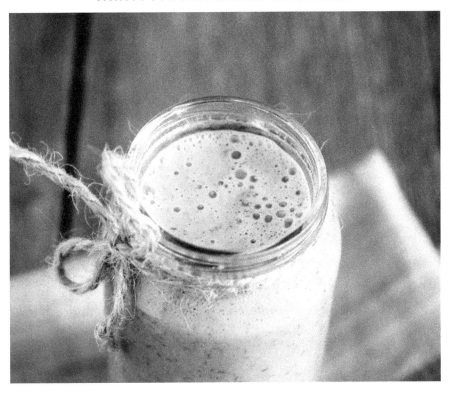

INGREDIENTS

3 cups spinach leaves

2 cups cubed ripe papaya 1 cup cubed pear

2 tablespoons goji berries (dried or fresh) 10 fresh leaves of mint

1 cup filtered water

DIRECTIONS

1. Pour water into blender. Add papaya first, followed by the

pear, berries and then mint

leaves. Add the spinach last.

2. Blend on high speed for about 30 seconds or until the smoothie turns into an even and creamy consistency.

3. Serve fresh.

Variation:

Substitute papaya with an equal part of banana and you will still have a creamy smoothie.

Pour smoothie into an airtight container and chill in the refrigerator overnight to make a refreshing morning smoothie meal replacement.

GREEN PIÑA COLADA SMOOTHIE

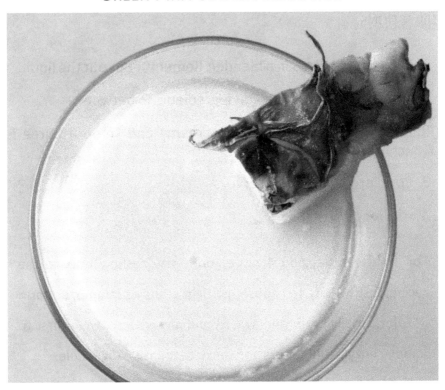

INGREDIENTS

- 1 cup chopped dandelion greens

- 4 cups fresh ripe pineapple chunks

- ½ cup shredded coconut meat 4 tablespoons dried pitted dates

- 2 cups unsweetened coconut water 2 cups ice cubes

DIRECTIONS

1. Put all ingredients in a blender. Remember to put the liquid first and the greens last. Add ingredients in between.

2. Blend on high speed until a creamy and smooth puree is achieved.

3. Pour into glasses and serve.

Variation:

For a nutty taste, add 4 tablespoons raw cashew nuts to the recipe. Just be sure to choose the right cashews (plump, uniform in color, smells nutty and sweet) and always soak them first to remove enzyme inhibitors and make them more digestible.

Kiwi Green Smoothie

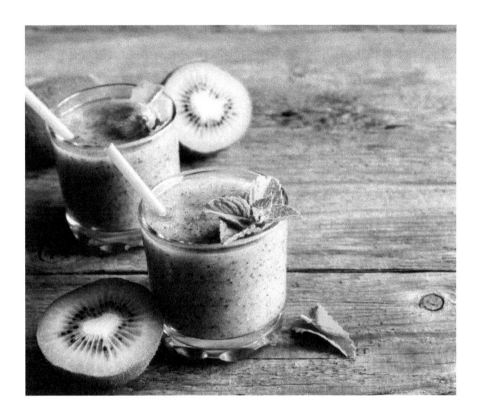

INGREDIENTS

- 1 cup chopped kale leaves
- 1 cup chopped Romaine lettuce
- 1 cup chopped Swiss chard leaves
- ½ cup sliced ripe bananas
- ½ kiwi fruit Juice of ½ lemon
- 1 cup distilled water 1 teaspoon bee pollen
- ½ teaspoon maca powder

DIRECTIONS

1. Wash all ingredients thoroughly. Prepare as directed in the recipe.

2. Put all ingredients in a blender. Blend at high speed until smooth.

3. Pour into a glass and serve immediately.

Variation:

Replace water with same amount of unsweetened coconut water for extra alkaline in your green smoothie. If kiwis are not in season, substitute it with mango or papaya.

MINTY GREEN SMOOTHIE

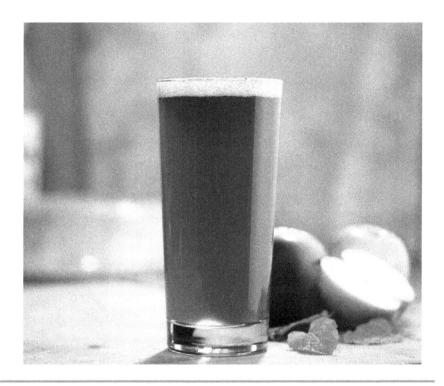

INGREDIENTS

- 1 cup chopped spinach leaves

- 10 pieces mint leaves

- 2 whole pitted dates

- 2 tablespoons raw cashew butter

- 1 ½ cups distilled water

DIRECTIONS

1. Put all ingredients in a blender. Whiz on high speed until smooth.

2. Pour into glasses and serve immediately.

Variation:

Substitute pitted dates with 1 tablespoon of raw coconut nectar or raw agave nectar Add 1 cup of ice cubes for a cold treat

Smoothie fact:

Mint not only triggers a feeling of satiety (it makes you feel full!) but also helps flush out toxins from the digestive tract. It also aids in proper digestion by soothing the intestines and loosening intestinal muscles, thus relieving cramps and other symptoms of disturbed stomach.

Avocado Lime Smoothie

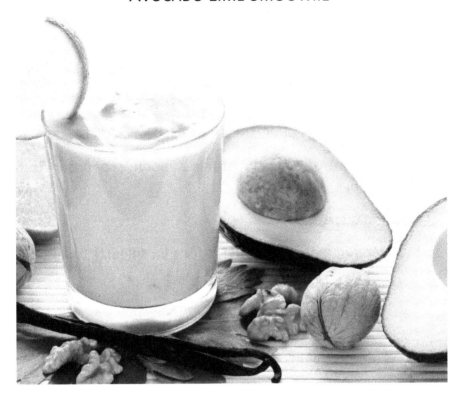

INGREDIENTS

- 1 cup spinach leaves

- ½ cup sliced cucmber

- ½ avocado fruit

- 6 pieces ice cubes

- 3 whole limes

- Sweetener (honey, agave or stevia) to taste

DIRECTIONS

1. Wash vegetables and fruits thoroughly.

2. Pluck out the leaves of the spinach. Discard stems.

3. Without peeling, cut cucumber into half-inch slices.

4. Remove seed of avocado. Using a spoon, scoop out flesh from the peeling.

5. Peel and quarter limes.

6. In a blender, place cucumber, avocado, spinach and lime.

Add ice cubes and desired

   amount of sweetener.

7. Blend all ingredients until smooth.

8. Pour into a glass and drink fresh.

Variation:

   Add ½ teaspoon cinnamon powder to add zing to your smoothie.

   If you find your smoothie too thick, add ½ cup of cold distilled water and blend again before serving.

Kale Green Smoothie

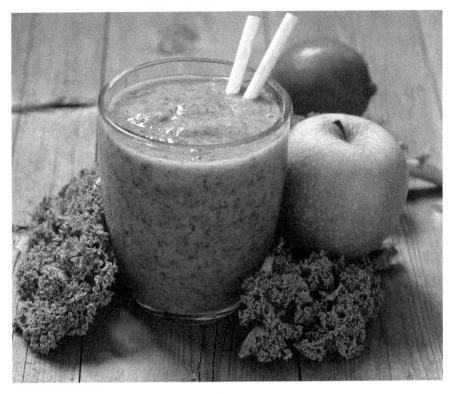

INGREDIENTS

- 1 cup kale leaves

- 1 medium sized apple

- 1 medium sized avocado

- ¼ lemon fruit

- 1 tablespoon sliced ginger

- A pinch of salt

- ½ cup distilled water

DIRECTIONS

1. Rinse kale in running water. Tear leaves apart.

2. Without peeling, core and segment apples.

3. Cut avocado into halves, remove seed and scoop out flesh using a tablespoon.

4. Peel lemon and remove seeds.

5. Peel ginger and cut into thin slices.

6. Put all ingredients in a blender. Whiz on high speed until well mixed and smooth.

7. Pour into a tall glass and enjoy!

Variation:

Use limes instead of lemon for a slightly different taste.

Instead of adding sweetener like honey or agave nectar, you can make this smoothie taste sweeter by adding more apples.

Instead of avocado, you can also use equal part banana in this recipe.

SUMMER SALAD SMOOTHIE

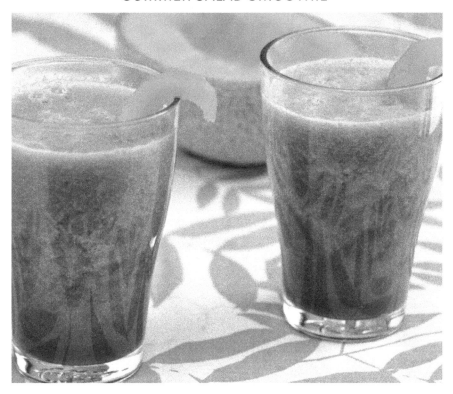

INGREDIENTS

- 10 leaves of mint
- 10 leaves of sweet basil
- 2 cups watermelon chunks
- ½ small avocado fruit
- ½ lime fruit
- ½ cup cucumber slices Juice of
- ½ cup distilled water
- 10 leaves of coriander

DIRECTIONS

1. Remove seeds from watermelon before cutting into chunks. Scoop out flesh from the

avocado fruit. Slice cucumbers into half-inch thickness.

2. Put all ingredients in a blender in this order: mint, basil, coriander, water, watermelon,

avocado, cucumber, lime juice. Blend on high speed until smooth.

3. Pour into a tall glass and serve.

Variation:

Add ½ teaspoon of fennel seeds and ½ cup oats for a more filling version of this smoothie. Put smoothie inside the freezer to cool it down for a few minutes before serving.

Detox Smoothie

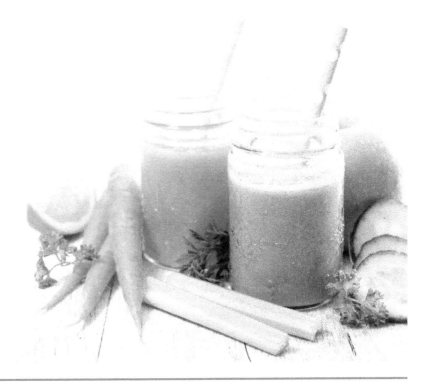

INGREDIENTS

- ½ cup broccoli heads

- 1 cup shredded romaine lettuce

- ½ orange

- ½ cup distilled water

- 1 cup ice cubes

- ½ orange

- ½ cup distilled water 1 cup ice cubes

DIRECTIONS

1. Rinse greens under running water.

2. Peel and core apple. Cut into 1-inch cubes.

3. Peel orange. Remove seeds and separate into segments.

4. Put all ingredients in a blender. Blend on high speed until thoroughly combined.

5. Pour into a glass and serve.

Variation:

Add 1 tablespoon of chopped parsley into the mix for added kick.

GINGER Smoothie

INGREDIENTS

- 1 cup spinach

- 1 cup figs (about 4 medium sized fruits)

- ½ tablespoon chopped ginger

- 2 whole pitted dates (pre-soaked)

- 1 cup ice cubes

- ½ cup distilled water DIRECTIONS

DIRECTIONS

1. In a blender, add spinach and water. Blend until smooth.

2. Add all remaining ingredients and process until blended smoothly.

3. Pour into a glass and enjoy.

Variation:

Add a tablespoon of flaxseeds for added zing.

Basic Banana Smoothie

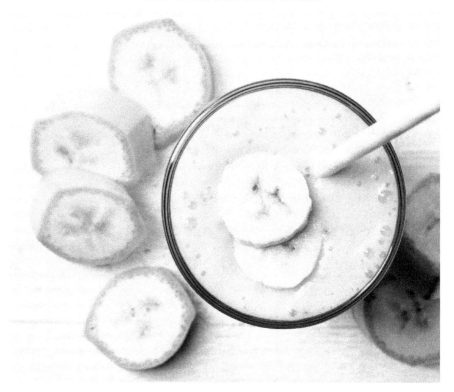

INGREDIENTS

- 2 cups diced ripe bananas
- 1 cup chopped kale leaves
- ½ cup distilled water
- ½ cup ice cubes.

1. Rinse kale in running water and clean thoroughly. 2. Peel bananas and cut into 1-inch slices.

3. Put all ingredients in a blender and whiz until smooth.

4. Pour into a glass and enjoy.

Variation:

For a sweeter taste, add 1 piece apple (cored and cut into wedges) into the recipe. This will infuse your smoothie with the toxin removal properties of apples.

ENERGIZER GREEN SMOOTHIE

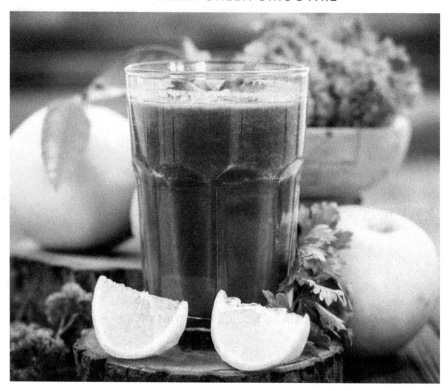

INGREDIENTS

- 2 pieces apples
- 1 piece banana
- 1 cup water
- ½ piece cucumber
- 1 kiwi

DIRECTIONS

1. Peel, core and cut apples into 1-inch cubes.

2. Peel banana and cut into 1-inch slices.

3. Without peeling, cut cucumbers into 1-inch cubes.

4. Place all ingredients in a blender and whiz until smooth.

5. Pour into a glass and serve immediately.

Variation:

To make a cold smoothie, use only ½ cup water and add ½ cup ice cubes. Blend well.

CACAO GREEN SMOOTHIE

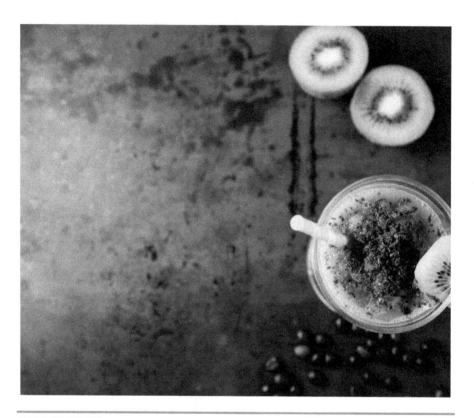

INGREDIENTS

- ½ cup chopped kale leaves
- 1 cup chopped romaine lettuce leaves
- ½ cup Swiss chard
- 1 cup sliced ripe bananas
- 1 teaspoon unsweetened cacao powder
- 1 tablespoon natural honey
- 1 cup unsweetened coconut water

- 1 Kiwi

DIRECTIONS

1. Rinse and prepare greens and fruits.

2. Peel bananas and cut into 1-inch slices.

3. Put all ingredients in a blender and process until smooth.

4. Pour into a glass and serve immediately.

Variation:

Add juice of ½ lemon for extra kick.

SUPER GREEN SMOOTHIE

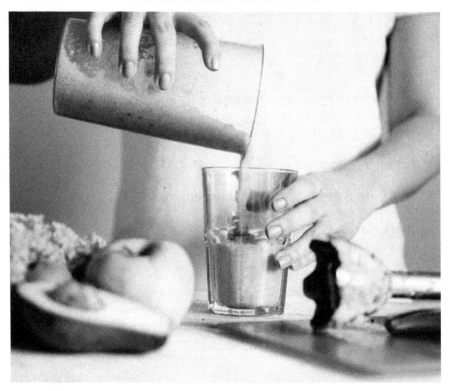

INGREDIENTS

- 1 cup chopped kale leaves
- ½ cup Brussels sprouts
- ½ cup spinach leaves
- ½ avocado
- 1 medium sized green apple
- ½ cup filtered water
- ½ cup ice cubes

DIRECTIONS

1. Wash and prepare the greens.

2. Scoop out the avocado flesh. Discard the seed.

3. Without peeling, core the apple and cut into 1-inch cubes.

4. In a blender, mix kale, Brussels sprouts, spinach and filtered water until smooth.

5. Add avocado, apple and ice cubes. Blend until smooth.

Variation:

Add 1 teaspoon chia seeds for an added punch

Add ½ cup broccoli or clover sprouts for extra greens

Mango and Celery Smoothie

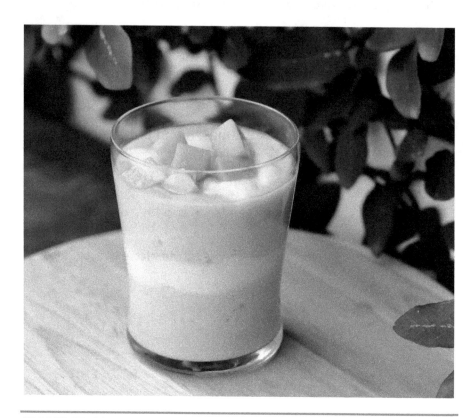

INGREDIENTS

- 1 cup chopped kale leaves

- ½ cup parsley leaves

- 1 medium stalk of celery

- ½ cup ripe mango chunks

- 1 cup coconut water

DIRECTIONS

1. Wash and prepare greens.

2. Cut celery stalk into 1-inch strips to facilitate easier blending.

3. Put all ingredients in a blender and mix until smooth.

4. Pour into a glass and enjoy.

Variation:

If mangoes are not in season, substitute with another fruit like pineapple or strawberry.

FRUITY GREEN SMOOTHIE

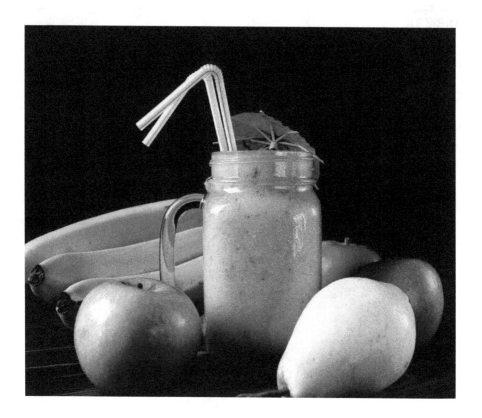

INGREDIENTS

- ½ cup chopped kale leaves
- ½ cup baby spinach leaves
- ½ cup raspberry or strawberry
- 1 cup sliced ripe banana
- 1 cup pear cubes
- 1 cup distilled water

DIRECTIONS

1. Pour water, kale and spinach in a blender. Whiz until smooth.

2. Add remaining ingredients and continue blending until smooth.

3. Pour into a glass and serve immediately.

Variation:

Top with a dash of cinnamon for an added kick.

If you want your smoothie cold, use only ½ cup of water and add ½ cup of ice cubes into the blend.

GREEN COCONUT SMOOTHIE

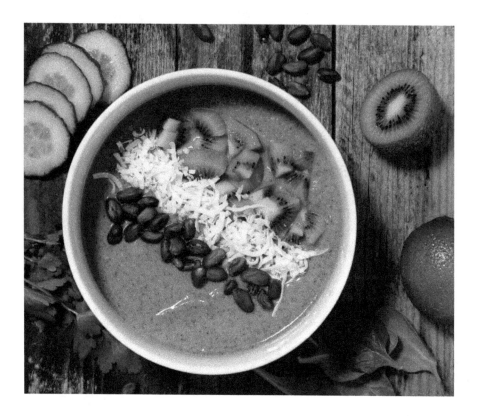

INGREDIENTS

- 1 teaspoon raw honey
- 1 cup sliced ripe bananas
- 1 cup chopped kale leaves
- 1 cup coconut meat
- 1 cup coconut water
- ½ cup ice cubes

DIRECTIONS

1. In a blender, mix all ingredients until smooth.

2. Pour into a glass and serve immediately.

Variation:

To make this smoothie even more nutritious, add 2 tablespoons of organic green barley powder and 1 tablespoon of chia seeds.

WILD BLUEBERRY KEFIR SMOOTHIE

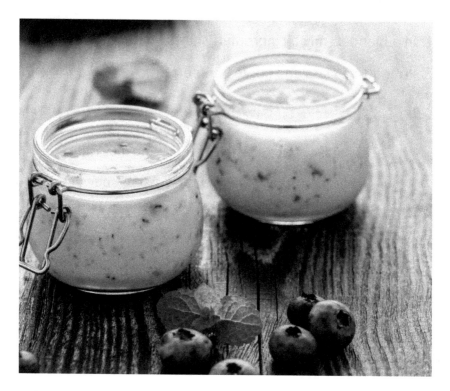

SERVINGS 2

INGREDIENTS

- 1½ cups frozen wild blueberries

- ¾ cup plain kefir

- ¾ cup whole milk yogurt (vanilla or a mix of plain and vanilla –Greek or regular)

- 2 tablespoons peanut butter

- 4 frozen spinach cubes (or 2 handfuls fresh baby spinach) optional: chia or hemp seeds

DIRECTIONS

- mix all ingredients in a blender and process until smooth

- add a little bit of water if needed to reach desired consistency

Nutrition *(per serving)Calories: 286; Total Fat: 14 g; SaturatedFat: 5 g; Protein: 13 g: Carbohydrates: 31 g;Sugar: 20 g; Fiber: 5 g;*

Cholesterol: 23 mg; Sodium: 202

Strawberry banana smoothie withspirulina

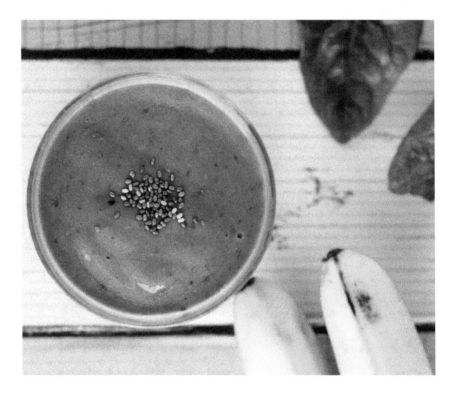

SERVINGS 1

INGREDIENTS

- 1 ripe banana
- 1/2 cup fresh strawberries
- 1 cup fresh baby spinach
- 1 teaspoon spirulina powder
- 1 tablespoon chia seeds

- 1 teaspoon vanilla extract

- 1 cup water

- 1 tablespoon honey or syrup (optional and to taste)

DIRECTIONS

- mix all ingredients in a blender until smooth and creamy

- add more water to make the smoothie thicker

Nutrition *(per serving) Calories: 180; Total Fat: 3 g; SaturatedFat: 0 g;*

Protein: 5 g: Carbohydrates: 38

GREEN DATE NUT SMOOTHIE

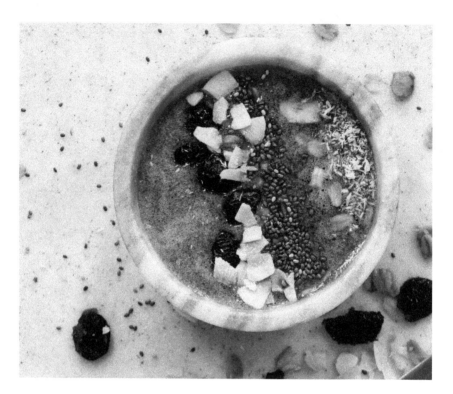

SERVINGS 2

INGREDIENTS

- 4 pitted dates (depending on size)

- 3 cups (packed) fresh spinach leaves

- 1 cup unsweetened almond milk

- 2 tablespoons almond butter

- 1 teaspoon ground cinnamon

- 1 cup ice

DIRECTIONS

- add 4 dates and the remaining ingredients into a blender.
- blend until smooth.
- taste, and add more dates if you'd like the smoothie to be a bit sweeter
- strain the mixture using a fine mesh strainer, and discard the remains
- serve cold

Nutrition *(per serving) Calories: 259; Total Fat: 10 g,Saturated Fat: 1 g; Protein: 7 g; Carbohydrates: 42 g*

MATCHA GREEN TEA SMOOTHIE

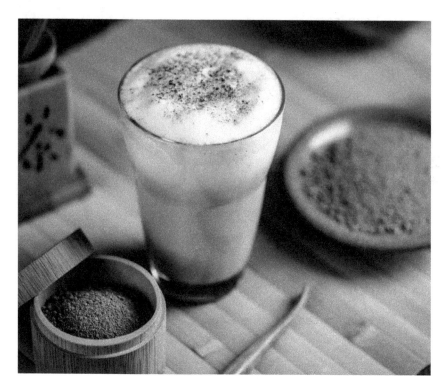

SERVINGS 1

INGREDIENTS

- 1½ teaspoons matcha powder

- 1 cup unsweetened vanilla almond milk

- 1 frozen banana

- 1 handful spinach

- 1 serving protein powder

- 1 cup ice

- 1 tablespoon chia seeds or 1/8 teaspoon xanthum gum, optional (provides volume)

DIRECTIONS

- place all ingredients into a blender and blend until smooth

Nutrition *(per serving) Calories: 264; Total Fat: 4 g; SaturatedFat: 0 g; Protein: 28 g; Carbohydrates: 32 g;*

GO GREEN SMOOTHIE

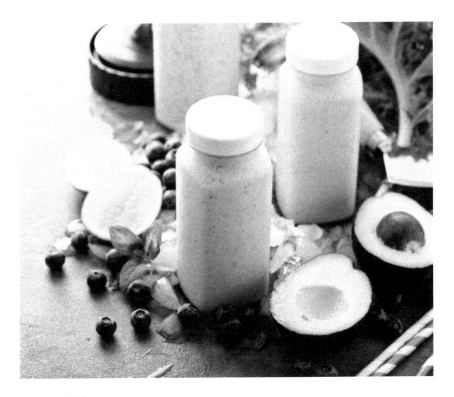

SERVINGS 2

INGREDIENTS

- 1 cup ice

- 1 medium banana, preferably frozen 2 scoops protein powderof choice

- 2-3 handfuls of spinach or greens of choice

- ½ avocado
- 1 ½-2 cups unsweetened almond milk or coconut milk

DIRECTIONS:

- place all ingredients into a blender in the order they are listedif using an upright blender

- blend until smooth and creamy and no chunks remain

- serve and enjoy (or store in a mason jar with lid for up to 24hours in the fridge)

Nutrition *(per serving) Calories: 215; Total Fat: 8 g; Protein: 13g; Carbohydrates: 22 g; Sugar: 7 g; Fiber: 7 g; Sodium: 180 mg*

ALMOND APPLE GREEN SMOOTHIE

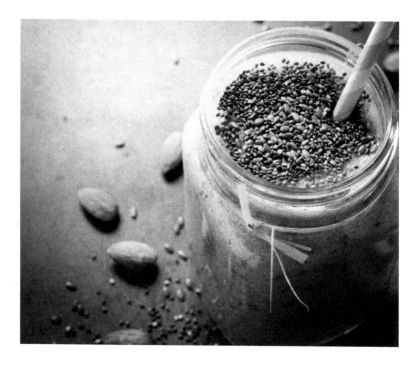

SERVINGS 1

INGREDIENTS

- 1 cup water
- 1/4 cup almonds raw, unsalted
- 2 stalks celery chopped into 2 inch cubes
- 1 handful spinach (about 1 cup)

70

- 1 medium apple, sliced

DIRECTIONS

- add water and almonds to your blender

- blend on high until the almonds start to break down

- add the celery, spinach and apple slices and blend until smooth

Nutrition *(per serving) Calories: 321; Total Fat: 18 g; SaturatedFat: 1 g; Protein: 9 g: Carbohydrates: 36 g; Sugar: 22 g; Fiber: 11 g;*

Cholesterol: 0 mg; Sodium: 97 mg

PEACH, BLUEBERRY AND SPINACH SMOOTHIE

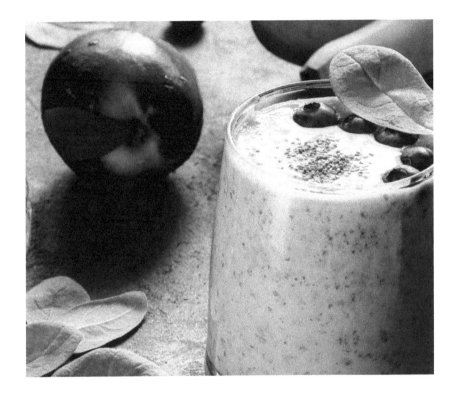

SERVINGS 1

INGREDIENTS

- ½ cup peaches

- ½ cup blueberries

- 2 cups spinach

- 1 scoops whey protein powder (I like Vanilla Gnarly Whey)

- 1 cup almond or coconut milk
- 1 cup ice

DIRECTIONS

- place all ingredients into a blender and blend until smooth

Nutrition *(per serving) Calories: 228; Total Fat: 4 g; SaturatedFat: 0 g; Protein: 29 g: Carbohydrates: 23 g;Sugar: 14 g; Fiber: 6 g;*

Cholesterol: 5 mg; Sodium: 278 mg

MANGO AND GREENS PICK-ME-UPSMOOTHIE

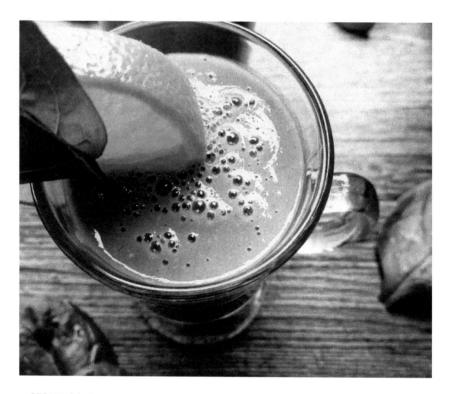

SERVINGS 2

INGREDIENTS

- 1 frozen banana

- 1 cup (packed) baby spinach

- 1 fresh mango, diced (about 1 cup)

- 1½ cups grass fed low fat milk or organic soy milk

DIRECTIONS

- place all ingredients in a blender and blend until smooth andserve

Nutrition *(per serving) Calories: 205; Total Fat: 2.3 g; Protein: 7.8g: Carbohydrates: 40 g; Fiber: 3.7 g; Cholesterol: 0 mg; Sodium: 95 mg*

PEACH AND WHITE BEAN SMOOTHIE

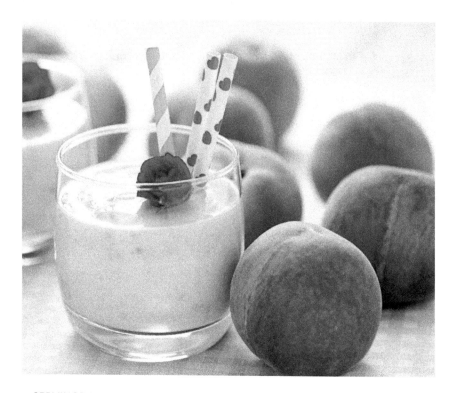

SERVINGS 1

INGREDIENTS

- ½ cup unsweetened rice milk

- 1 cup frozen peaches

- ¼ cup canned white beans (like cannellini, navy or great northern)

- 1/8 teaspoon cinnamon
- pinch of nutmeg

DIRECTIONS

- pour the rice milk into the blender
- add the remaining ingredients and blend until smooth

Nutrition *(per serving) Calories394.1g; Total Fat16.4 g; Saturated Fat1.9 g; Polyunsaturated Fat3.5 g; Monounsaturated Fat9.9g; Cholesterol4.3 mg; Sodium298.3 mg; Potassium1,174.9 mg; Total Carbohydrate47.2 g; Dietary Fiber11.1 g; Sugars19.0 g; Protein19.9 g*

BELLY FAT BURNING SMOOTHIE

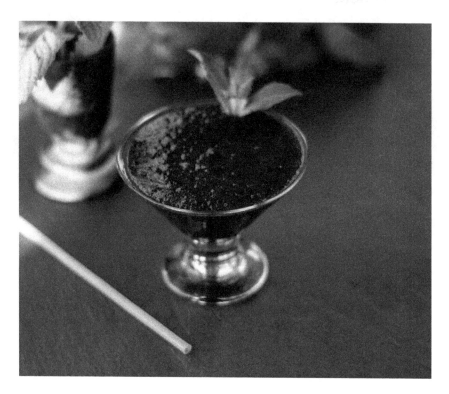

SERVINGS 1

INGREDIENTS

- ½ avocado
- ¼ cup Greek yogurt
- ½ cup of pomegranate juice
- ½ tablespoon honey
- ½ teaspoon vanilla extract
- ½ cup ice
- 1 tablespoon whey protein

DIRECTIONS

- put all ingredients in blender and blend to your desired smoothness
- Whey protein helps build muscle which helps you to burn calories

Nutrition *(per serving)* *Calories 300g; Total Fat1g; SaturatedFat1.9 g; Polyunsaturated Fat3.5 g; Monounsaturated Fat 9.9 g; Cholesterol1.3 mg; Sodium298.3 mg; Potassium1,174.9 mg; Total Carbohydrate 36.2 g; Dietary Fiber 16.1 g; Sugars16.0 g; Protein 15.9 g*

GLEAMING GREEN SPINACH AND

LETTUCE SMOOTHIE

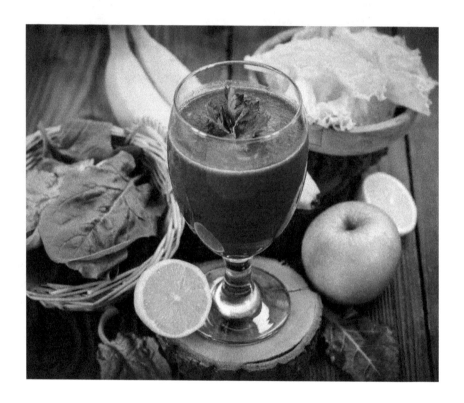

SERVINGS 2

INGREDIENTS

- 3 cups chopped romaine lettuce (or about 1 head)
- 2 cups chopped spinach leaves (about half of a large bunch)
- ½ cup sliced celery
- ½ cup diced apples (about ½ medium sized whole)
- ¼ cup diced pear (about 1 medium sized wholes)
- ½ cup sliced banana
- ½ tablespoon fresh lemon juice
- 1 cup water

DIRECTIONS

- put lettuce, spinach and water together in a blender
- process at low speed until mixture becomes smooth
- add celery, apple and pear
- blend mixture at high speed
- lastly, add the banana and lemon juice and puree until well blended
- pour into glasses and serve fresh

Nutrition *(per serving) Calories 198 g; Total Fat 10g; Saturated Fat 1g; Total Carbohydrate 47 g; Dietary Fiber 5 g; Sugars 40 g; Protein 59g*

ENERGY BOOSTER SPINACH AND COLLARDGREENS

SMOOTHIE

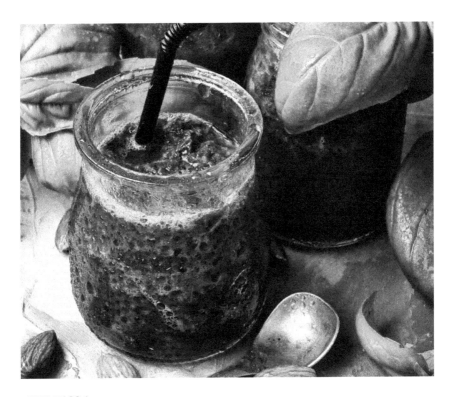

SERVINGS 1

INGREDIENTS

- 1cup fresh spinach
- 1cup fresh collard greens
- 4whole medium sized oranges
- 3cups pineapple chunks

DIRECTIONS

- squeeze out the juice from the oranges
- use this fresh juice as liquid base for blending the spinach and collard greens together
- blend at slow speed until smooth
- add the pineapples to the orange and greens mixture andblend at high speed until well mixed
- pour and serve immediately

Nutrition (*per serving*) *Calories 163 g; Total Fat 2g; Saturated Fat 0g; Total Carbohydrate 36 g; Dietary Fiber 5 g; Sugars 26 g; Protein 3 g*

Minty Papaya Green Smoothie

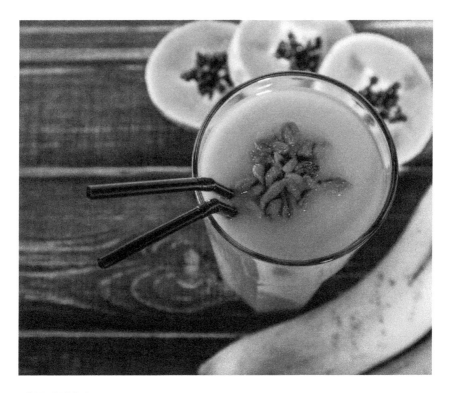

SERVINGS 1

INGREDIENTS

- 3 cups spinach leaves

- 2 cups cubed ripe papaya

- 1 cup cubed pear

- 2 tablespoons goji berries (dried or fresh)

- 10 fresh leaves of mint

- 1 cup filtered water

DIRECTIONS

- pour water into blender.

- add papaya first, followed by the pear, berries and then mint leaves, add the spinach last

- blend on high speed for about 30 seconds or until the smoothie turns into an even and creamy consistency

- serve fresh

Nutrition (*per serving*) *Calories 126 g; Total Fat 0.1g; Saturated Fat 0g; Total Carbohydrate 27.8 g; Dietary Fiber 2.4 g; Sugars 15 g; Protein*

5.1 g

GRAPEFRUIT PINEAPPLE SPLASH

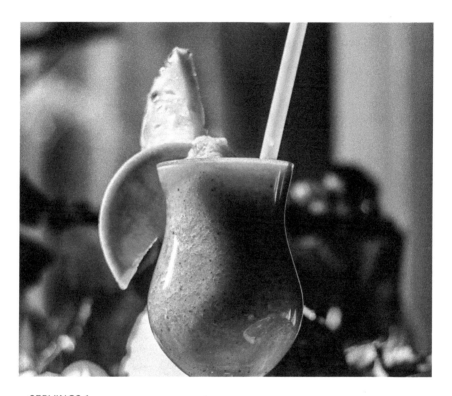

SERVINGS 1

6

INGREDIENTS

- 2 medium pink grapefruit
- 2 small pineapples
- 1 ½ cups sparkling water
- 5 ice cubes

DIRECTIONS

- peel the grapefruit and pineapple, removing any seeds and the pineapple core
- chop the pineapple into large pieces
- put both fruits, the sparkling water and the ice cubes into a powerful blender
- process until the result is smooth and bubbly

Nutrition *(per serving) Calories: 271g; Carbohydrates:*

46g; Protein: 8g; Fat:8g; Saturated Fat: 0g; Fiber: 13g; Sugar: 25g

Tasty Cashew Shake

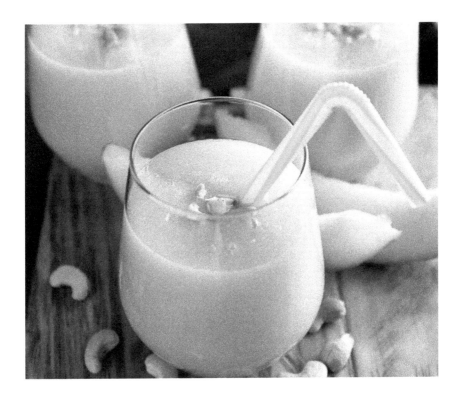

SERVING 1

INGREDIENTS

- ½ cup whole raw cashews or almonds
- ¼ cup whole strawberries
- 1 small vanilla bean
- ½ teaspoon cinnamon

- 5 ice cubes

DIRECTIONS

- soak the cashews for one hour in one cup of water to softenthem and make them easier to blend
- hull the strawberries, discarding the leaves
- combine the cashews, their soaking water, and all other ingredients in a powerful blender on high
- process until the mixture is smooth and frothy

Nutrition (per serving)) *Calories 326 g; Total Fat 19g; Saturated Fat 3g; Total Carbohydrate 80 g; Dietary Fiber 7 g; Sugars 57 g; Protein 9 g*

BANANA AVOCADO GREEN SMOOTHIE

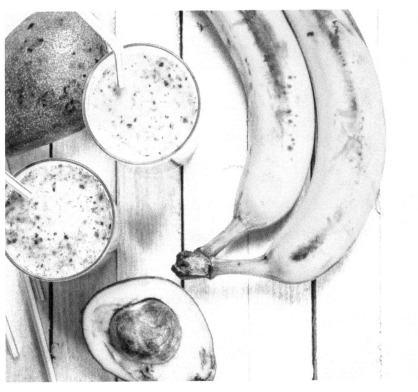

INGREDIENTS

- 1 cup Swiss chard leaves
- 1 cup unripe banana chunks
- 1 cup spinach
- ½ medium sized cucumber
- ½ avocado
- 1 whole lime
- ½ cup young coconut meat

- 1 cup unsweetened coconut water

DIRECTIONS

1. Wash spinach, Swiss chard and cucumber thoroughly in running water. Chop the leaves and cut the cucumber into 1-inch cubes.

2. Peel bananas and cut into 1-inch slices.

3. Scoop out the flesh of the avocado. Discard the seed.

4. Peel the lime and quarter.

5. In a blender, mix spinach, Swiss chard and coconut water until smooth.

6. Add remaining ingredients and blend until smooth and mixed thoroughly.

Variation:

Add 3-5 mint leaves into the blend for an added punch and cooling effect. If you want your smoothie cold, chill in the refrigerator before drinking. To sweeten smoothie, add a bit of honey or mix a medium sized cored and cubed red apple when blending.

TROPICAL GREEN KALE SMOOTHIE

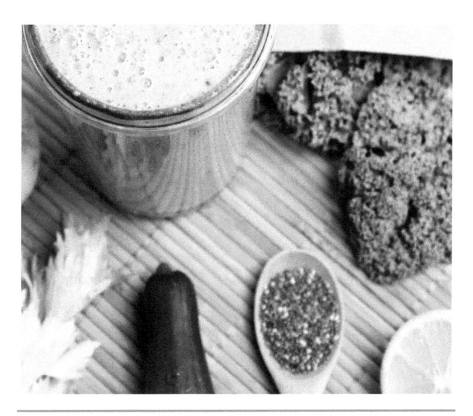

INGREDIENTS

- 3 cups chopped kale leaves

- 1 whole medium sized mango

- ½ cup sliced banana

- ½ lime fruit

- cup unsweetened coconut milk

DIRECTIONS

1. Wash and prepare all ingredients. Peel the mango, remove the seed and slice into 2-inch cubes. Juice the lime fruit.

2. Pour coconut milk into blender. Add mango, banana and lime juice. Add kale leaves last.

3. Blend all ingredients on high speed until smoothie reaches a creamy consistency (This will take about 30 seconds to process).

4. Pour into a glass and serve fresh.

Variation:

Serve chilled or over crushed ice for a refreshing drink perfect during hot days. Do without the ice but use chilled or frozen chunks of mangoes instead. For a surprisingly cool twist, do not puree the mangoes and just add the mango chunks just before serving.

SPINACH YOGURT SMOOTHIE

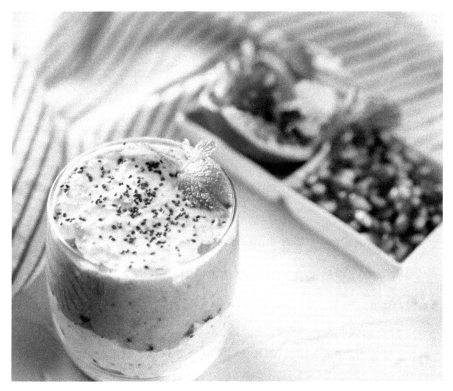

INGREDIENTS

- 2 cups chopped spinach leaves

- 1 large whole orange

- ½ cup sliced bananas

- 1/3 cup strawberries

- 1/3 cup plain yogurt
- 1 cup ice cubes

DIRECTIONS

1. Peel oranges and divide into segments. Remove seeds if there are any.
2. Put all ingredients in a blender. Puree until smooth.
3. Pour into glasses and serve immediately.

Variation:

Although this recipe calls for strawberries, you can use other kinds of berries, too. Be not afraid, experiment!

Mango Smoothie Surprise

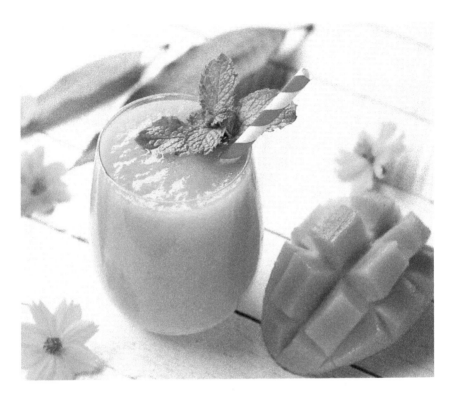

SERVINGS: 1

INGREDIENTS

- ¼ cup mango cubes
- ¼ cup mashed ripe avocado (MUFA)

- ½ cup mango juice

- ¼ cup fat-free vanilla yogurt

- 1 tbsp freshly squeezed lime juice 1 Tbsp sugar

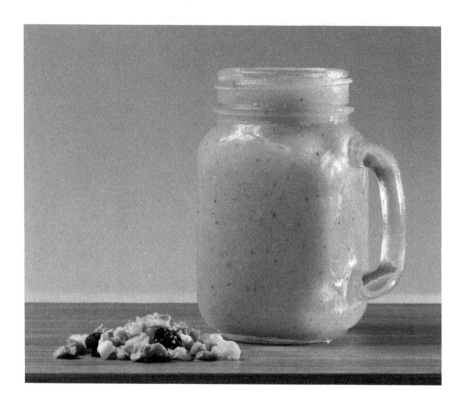

- 6 ice cubes

DIRECTIONS

- place all ingredients in a blender and process until smooth
- pour into a tall glass and garnish with sliced mango or strawberry, if desired, and serve

-

Nutrition *(per serving) 298 cal, 5 g pro, 55 g carb, 5 g fiber, 47 gsugar, 9 g fat, 1.5 g sat fat, 54 mg sodi*

PEACHY GREEN SMOOTHIE

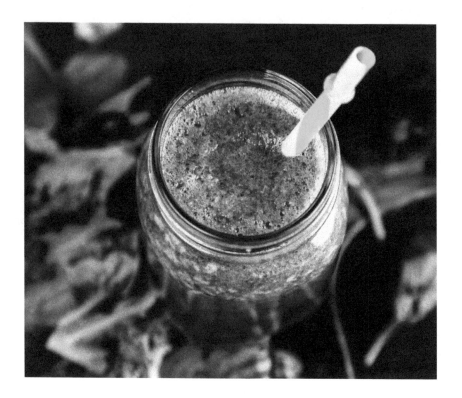

SERVINGS 1

INGREDIENTS

- 1 peach
- 1 banana
- 1 cup of kale
- 1 scoop of whey protein

- 6 frozen strawberries

- Almond milk as needed

- Ice cubes

DIRECTIONS

- place all ingredients into the blender container in the order listed and secure the lid

- start the blender on its lowest speed, then quickly increase to its highest speed

- blend for 30-45 seconds or until desired consistency is reached, using the tamper to press ingredients toward the blades

Nutrition *(per serving) Calories 197 g; Total Fat 5g; Saturated Fat 1g; Total Carbohydrate 37 g; Dietary Fiber 8g; Sugars 23g; Protein 5g*

WATERMELON SMOOTHIE

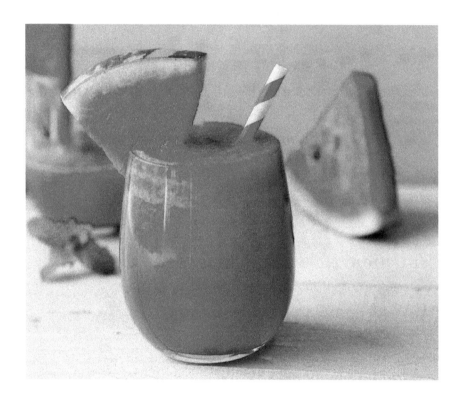

SERVINGS 1

INGREDIENTS

- 6 cups of seedless watermelon
- 1 cup of lemon sherbet
- 6 ice cubes
- 1 cup frozen strawberries
- ½ cup vanilla Greek yogurt
- 1/2 tablespoon honey

DIRECTIONS

- place all ingredients in a high-powered blender
- blend until smooth, adding more water as needed if the smoothie is too thick
- taste and add additional honey if you'd like the smoothie sweeter

Nutrition *(per serving) Calories 157 g; Total Fat 1g; Saturated Fat 1g; Total Carbohydrate 35 g; Dietary Fiber 3g; Sugars 29g; Protein 7g*

ACAI BERRY BLASTER

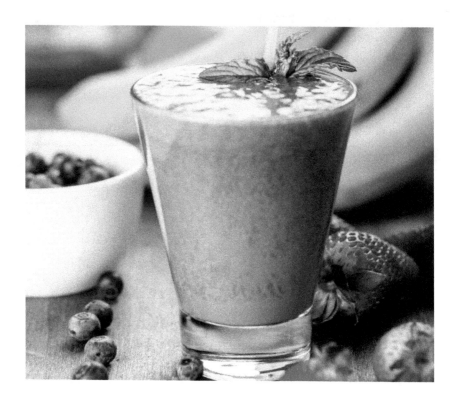

SERVINGS 1

INGREDIENTS

- ¼ cup acai berry puree 1½ cup strawberries
- ¾ cup blueberries
- 1 small banana, peeled and split into pieces 1 tablespoon pure cacao powder
- 1 cup non-dairy milk

DIRECTIONS

- carefully add all of the ingredients into the blender and pulse on medium powder until all of the ingredients have been combined and the mixture is smooth

Nutrition *(per serving) Calories 201 g; Total Fat 3g; Saturated Fat 1g; Total Carbohydrate 45g; Dietary Fiber 3g; Sugars 29g; Protein 3g*

MOCHA SMOOTHIE

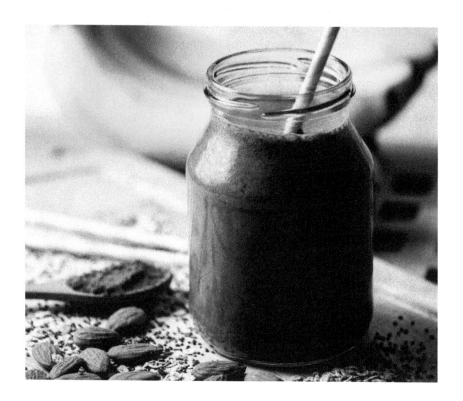

SERVINGS 1

INGREDIENTS

- ½ cup of low-fat vanilla yogurt
- 1 shot of espresso
- 2 teaspoons of cocoa powder
- Almond milk as needed
- 4 small ice cubes

DIRECTIONS

- add all the ingredients to a blender and blend until smooth
- pour into a glass and enjoy

Nutrition *(per serving) Calories 369 g; Total Fat 3g; Saturated Fat 1g; Total Carbohydrate 57 g; Dietary Fiber 4g; Sugars 40g; Protein 30g*